THE

DIABETES

CODE FOR SENIORS

Embracing Diabetes in the Golden Years

By

Dr. Andrew Morrison

TABLE OF CONTENTS

EMOTIONAL WELL-BEING AND COPING MECHANISMS
ESTABLISHING A NETWORK OF SUPPORT FOR MENTAL HEALTH
DIABETES COPING TECHNIQUES AND MENTAL HEALTH NURTURING

<u>CONCLUSION</u>

INTRODUCTION

COMPREHENDING DIABETES IN SENIORS

Chronic metabolic disorders like diabetes provide unique problems for older people navigating their golden years. This book explores the intricacies of diabetes in the older population, including its kinds, prevalence, risk factors, and effective management strategies in light of aging.

The prevalence of diabetes rises dramatically with age. Studies indicate that a sizable proportion of older persons may have prediabetes or diabetes, highlighting the need to comprehend and treat this health issue in the aging population.

Different forms of diabetes can affect older people, with type 2 diabetes being the most prevalent. This variety frequently appears later in life and is impacted by aging itself, genetics, and lifestyle choices. Some elderly people who have had Type 1 diabetes since childhood can still manage it.

Older people are more likely to develop diabetes due to a number of variables. These include modifications in metabolism brought on by aging, as well as possible weight gain, a decline in physical activity, and the long-term effects of lifestyle decisions. It is essential to comprehend these risk factors in order to prevent problems and effectively manage them.

Taking care of diabetes presents special difficulties for senior citizens. The treatment approach may become more complicated if there are coexisting medical disorders, such as cognitive impairment or cardiovascular problems. Furthermore, in order to prevent any interactions, factors like polypharmacy—the practice of people taking multiple medications for different conditions—need to be carefully considered.

Diabetes in older people frequently calls for a customized approach to drug administration. The selection of pharmaceuticals ought to take into consideration the specific medical issues of the elderly person, possible adverse effects, and their general state of health. It takes regular observation and correction to keep blood sugar levels at their ideal levels.

CHAPTER ONE

DIETARY GUIDELINES FOR DIABETES IN OLDER ADULTS

An important aspect of managing diabetes in older people is meeting their nutritional needs. It's crucial to prepare balanced meals that take dietary limitations, possible dental problems, and appetite fluctuations into account. Additionally, paying attention to nutritional consumption becomes increasingly crucial to maintaining general health and well-being.

Maintaining an active lifestyle is essential for older people with diabetes. It becomes crucial to modify exercise regimens to account for aging bodies, consider joint health, and include activities that improve balance. Frequent exercise promotes general cardiovascular health in addition to aiding in blood sugar regulation.

The management of diabetes in older people necessitates periodic blood sugar monitoring and check-ups. Medical practitioners are able to modify treatment regimens, spot possible issues early on, and offer advice on changing one's lifestyle. Getting regular medical care is essential to preserving good health throughout old age.

It's important to acknowledge the emotional toll that diabetes has on older people. Stress and emotional strain can be exacerbated by age, managing a chronic illness, and other lifestyle changes. Comprehensive diabetes care requires an understanding of these emotional factors and the management of them.

An extensive support system is very beneficial to older people as they navigate the process of managing diabetes. Support groups, medical professionals, family, and friends are all important components of a comprehensive treatment plan. Emotional support, emotional support, and open communication create a supportive environment that helps older adults with diabetes manage their condition well.

A comprehensive strategy that takes into account the particular difficulties and factors associated with aging is necessary to comprehend diabetes in older people. With an understanding of the types, prevalence, and risk factors, along with individualized approaches to nutrition, medicine, and mental health, older people can manage their diabetes journey with empowerment and knowledge-based decision-making.

Handling the Particular Difficulties of Aging with Diabetes

The human body undergoes several changes as we age, and those who have diabetes face particular difficulties that must be carefully navigated. This article examines the unique problems that older people with diabetes have, providing information on health-related difficulties, lifestyle modifications, and management techniques that work as they age.

Physiological changes associated with aging affect the body's glucose regulation. As insulin resistance rises, blood sugar regulation becomes increasingly difficult. The pancreas may also generate less insulin, which would make managing diabetes even more difficult. Developing effective treatment regimens requires an understanding of these age-related changes.

Diabetes in older people frequently coexists with other medical disorders. Diabetes may coexist with conditions like cardiovascular disease, kidney disease, or cognitive loss, requiring an all-encompassing approach to healthcare. To treat the interplay of these disorders and maximize general health, coordinated management is essential.

Older people frequently use many medications at the same time, a condition known as polypharmacy. In order to prevent interactions and negative effects, managing diabetes while taking medication for other health conditions takes careful thought. In order to guarantee the best possible health outcomes and simplify pharmaceutical regimens, cooperation among healthcare providers is essential.

Diabetes self-care is complicated by the cognitive deterioration that comes with age. It could get harder to remember prescription regimens, check blood sugar levels, and follow dietary advice. Adopting techniques like reminders, medication organizers, and caregiver involvement can help people stick to regular self-care schedules.

Dietary choices, appetite, and digestion can all alter as we age. Nutritional difficulties, like trouble chewing or reduced taste sensitivity, can influence what you eat. It becomes essential to create diabetic-friendly recipes that take these things into account. Dietary programs can be specifically tailored to the needs of older people with diabetes by working with a nutritionist.

While staying physically active is essential for managing diabetes, aging can cause problems with mobility. Joint issues, a decline in muscle mass, or balance issues may restrict options for exercise. Promoting physical well-being requires adapting exercise regimens to these changes, including low-impact activities, and emphasizing flexibility and balancing exercises.

The cornerstone of managing diabetes is still routine blood sugar monitoring, yet older people may find it difficult to use conventional monitoring equipment. Technological innovations can improve accessibility; examples are glucose meters with larger screens and more user-friendly features. For self-monitoring to be effective, training and continuing assistance are essential.

Older folks frequently worry about social isolation, and those who have diabetes may be more vulnerable. Insufficient social contact can have an effect on mental health by making stress and depression more likely. Creating and sustaining a robust social support system, engaging in community events, and pursuing mental health assistance are essential elements of comprehensive diabetes management.

As one ages, navigating the financial side of healthcare becomes increasingly important. Diabetes patients may have higher healthcare costs, particularly if they are also managing other medical issues. These issues can be resolved by being aware of insurance coverage, looking into aid options, and being upfront and honest with healthcare professionals about financial limitations.

Planning for death is an essential part of aging with diabetes. It is ensured that patients receive treatment that is consistent with their beliefs by having conversations about their choices for care, creating advance directives, and sharing these requests with family members and medical professionals. An individualized and respectful approach to care is supported when diabetes treatment is included in end-of-life planning.

Managing the particular difficulties of aging while living with diabetes calls for a comprehensive and customized strategy. Through the management of physiological changes, the integration of treatment for coexisting illnesses, and the adoption of self-care, nutrition, and mental health initiatives, older persons with diabetes can effectively navigate their diabetes journey and sustain optimal well-being well into old age.

Encouraging a Positive Attitude to Handle Diabetes

Diabetes has a significant impact on mental and emotional health in addition to physical health, making living with the disease a lifelong adventure. For those with diabetes, having an optimistic outlook is essential because it enables them to overcome obstacles, make wise decisions, and promote general well-being. This article discusses methods for cultivating optimism in the face of the challenges associated with managing diabetes.

Building a happy mentality begins with acknowledging the connection between the mind and body. Diabetes management entails understanding the influence of emotions, stress, and mental outlook on physical health, in addition to tracking blood sugar levels and following medication regimens.

An effective tool for managing diabetes is knowledge. Giving people thorough knowledge about their illness, available treatments, and lifestyle options fosters confidence and a sense of control. Education reduces the uncertainty and anxiety associated with diabetes by acting as a catalyst for educated decision-making.

Maintaining long-term diabetes control requires adopting new lifestyle habits with optimism. People can reframe dietary changes, exercise regimens, and medication adherence as opportunities for self-care, well-being, and improved quality of life instead of seeing them as limitations.

Setting and achieving attainable goals is essential to keeping a good outlook. Establishing tiny, achievable goals, whether they have to do with food, exercise, or blood sugar targets, makes one feel accomplished. Honouring these successes, no matter how small, helps one maintain a positive perspective on their journey with diabetes.

Creating and maintaining a solid support system is essential to cultivating an optimistic outlook. Support groups, medical professionals, friends, and family can offer empathy, encouragement, and a feeling of belonging. A friendly atmosphere that fosters open communication and experience sharing has a favourable impact on mental health.

Deep breathing exercises and other mindfulness techniques are useful strategies for reducing diabetes-related stress. These techniques improve emotional resilience, lessen anxiety, and foster present-moment awareness. Including mindfulness in everyday activities helps cultivate a more upbeat and focused mind-set.

Diabetes can cause a wide range of emotions, such as loneliness, worry, and frustration. The first step in resolving these emotional difficulties is acknowledging them. Emotional well-being is enhanced by joining diabetes support groups, seeking professional mental health assistance, and expressing emotions honestly.

Maintaining a healthy weight requires physical activity, and adding fun things to your routine makes exercise even more beneficial. Taking part in joyful hobbies, such as dance, gardening, or leisurely walks, helps to foster a happy outlook and promotes regular physical activity.

It is imperative for people with diabetes to cultivate a healthy relationship with food. Embracing a varied and balanced approach to meals promotes enjoyment and satisfaction rather than seeing dietary limits as limitations. A good meal experience is enhanced by experimenting with different flavours, recipes, and mindful eating techniques.

There will inevitably be difficulties and setbacks while you have diabetes. Developing resilience and self-compassion are key components of cultivating a positive outlook. A resilient and optimistic mind-set is facilitated by acknowledging that each person's path with diabetes is different, forgiving oneself for moments of incompetence, and overcoming obstacles head-on.

Promoting a good outlook for diabetes management is an ongoing, life-changing endeavour. People can thrive on their diabetes journey by embracing information, setting realistic objectives, creating supporting networks, and placing a high priority on their mental health. Maintaining a positive outlook not only makes treating diabetes easier, but it also promotes general health and a happy existence.

CHAPTER TWO

CUSTOMIZING FOOD TO MANAGE DIABETES OPTIMALLY

Seniors managing diabetes need to pay close attention to their diet. Dietary requirements change as people age, and for those who have diabetes, it's critical to comprehend how meal choices affect blood sugar levels. This article explores the complex interplay between nutrition and the management of diabetes in the elderly, offering advice on meal planning, dietary restrictions, and health-promoting techniques.

The main objective of diabetes management for the elderly is to maintain stable blood sugar levels. It's critical to balance the three macronutrients: lipids, proteins, and carbohydrates. Since carbohydrates have a direct effect on blood sugar, it is best to spread them out throughout the day to avoid blood sugar spikes. Lean protein and good fats are important components of a balanced diet.

Understanding a food's glycaemic load (GL) and glycaemic index (GI) is beneficial for senior citizens with diabetes. The GI calculates the rate at which a food raises blood sugar, whereas the

GL takes into account the quantity and quality of carbs. Selecting foods with low GI and low GL helps improve blood sugar regulation.

In order to control their calorie intake and prevent overtaxing their digestive systems, seniors should exercise portion control. Snacks and smaller, more balanced meals spaced out throughout the day can help control blood sugar levels. Timing meals consistently helps seniors with diabetes maintain regular blood sugar management.

Seniors with diabetes must include foods high in fibre in their diet. Fibre facilitates digestion, reduces the rate at which sugar is absorbed, and helps keep blood sugar levels stable. Legumes, fruits, vegetables, and whole grains are excellent sources of dietary fibre that support a healthy digestive system and general wellbeing.

Foods high in nutrients offer vital vitamins and minerals without being overly caloric or sweetened. Diets high in nutrients, such as leafy greens, colourful vegetables, lean proteins, and fatty fish, should be given priority by seniors with diabetes. These meals help satisfy dietary requirements and promote general health without interfering with blood sugar regulation.

Individualized meal planning that takes into account their particular dietary preferences, medical problems, and lifestyle is beneficial for seniors with diabetes. Working together with a qualified dietitian makes it easier to develop customized meal plans that take individual preferences and tastes into account while meeting certain nutritional needs.

Seniors with diabetes need to drink enough water. Maintaining adequate hydration facilitates digestion, maintains renal function, and helps control blood sugar levels. Throughout the day, seniors should try to balance their intake of water and other sugar-free, non-caffeinated beverages.

Diabetes in older adults frequently increases the risk of cardiovascular problems. It is essential to monitor salt consumption in order to control blood pressure and maintain general cardiovascular health. Making flavourful substitutions with low-sodium options and adding herbs and spices improves heart health without sacrificing diabetic care.

Personalized diet plans are essential for elderly diabetics. Dietary decisions may be impacted by age-related concerns, such as metabolic changes and probable dental problems. Seniors may need to make changes to their diet plan based on their overall health, digestion, and dental comfort.

To get the best nutritional treatment possible, seniors with diabetes should work with medical specialists, such as registered dietitians and healthcare practitioners. A complete approach to senior diabetes treatment includes regular monitoring, meal plan modifications depending on health changes, and ongoing guidance.

Nutrition has a multifaceted role in the management of elders with diabetes, affecting not only blood sugar regulation but also general health and wellbeing. Through the adoption of a balanced macronutrient diet, knowledge of the glycaemic index, emphasis on nutrient-dense foods, and customization of meal planning, seniors can effectively manage their diabetic condition while maintaining optimal health and vigour.

Creating Well-Balanced Meals to Manage Blood Sugar

For those who are controlling their diabetes, eating balanced meals is essential to maintaining good blood sugar control. Creating meals that balance blood sugar levels and maximize nutrition is essential for general health and well-being. The fundamentals of preparing balanced meals that assist blood sugar regulation are examined in this article, which also provides information on food selections, portion sizes, and meal planning techniques.

In order to keep blood sugar levels steady, people with diabetes must balance their meals. Maintaining equilibrium among macronutrients, namely carbs, proteins, and fats, guarantees a consistent energy source for the body while reducing variations in blood glucose levels.

Since carbohydrates directly affect blood sugar, controlling them is an important part of meal planning. Long-term blood sugar stability is supported by selecting complex carbohydrates with a low glycaemic index (GI), such as legumes, whole grains, and non-starchy vegetables.

Meals containing lean proteins are essential for maintaining energy levels and encouraging fullness. Lean protein sources like chicken, fish, tofu, lentils, and low-fat dairy provide important amino acids without significantly raising blood sugar levels.

Including good fats in meals promotes nutrition absorption and increases feelings of fullness. Sources of healthful fats include avocados, almonds, seeds, and olive oil. Consuming these fats in moderation improves cardiovascular health overall and helps to normalize blood sugar levels.

In addition to helping to maintain digestive health, fibre is essential for controlling blood sugar levels. Including foods high in fibre, such as legumes, whole grains, fruits, and vegetables, slows down the absorption of glucose and promotes a sensation of fullness.

To prevent overburdening the digestive system and triggering abrupt rises in blood sugar, portion control is crucial. Using smaller plates, measuring quantities, and paying attention to serving sizes all help to better regulate blood sugar levels after meals.

Having meals spaced out throughout the day helps maintain stable blood sugar control. Snacking in between meals reduces the chance of hypoglycaemia and helps avoid prolonged periods without eating. This is an alternative to relying solely on three substantial meals.

Blood sugar levels are influenced by meal timing, highlighting the significance of regularity. Timing meals consistently encourages stable blood sugar levels by assisting the body in anticipating the availability of nutrients. Blood sugar responses are more predictable when meals and snacks are consumed on a regular basis.

Achieving balance involves more than just the total amount consumed each day; it also involves the makeup of each meal. A balanced meal that includes a combination of carbohydrates, proteins, and fats gives you long-lasting energy and helps you maintain ideal blood sugar levels all day.

Different people react differently to eating, which emphasizes the significance of routinely checking blood sugar levels. By observing the effects of several meals on blood glucose levels, people can modify their meal plans with knowledge and spot trends that promote the best possible blood sugar control.

A proactive and powerful strategy for managing diabetes is to prepare healthy meals specifically designed to control blood sugar levels. Through the prioritization of nutrient-dense foods, prudent management of carbs, the incorporation of lean proteins and healthy fats, and portion control, people can make confident dietary choices that support stable blood sugar levels and promote overall well-being.

Dealing with Dietary Issues Particular to Elderly People

Dietary needs and problems change with age, and it is especially important for older adults with diabetes to take these particular dietary factors into account. The special dietary needs of elderly people with diabetes are examined in this article, which also provides information on age-related changes, potential roadblocks, and useful tips for promoting healthy eating and blood sugar management.

Aging is related to natural metabolic changes that might alter how the body uses nutrients, particularly glucose. Diabetes in older adults may result in a reduction in insulin sensitivity, which makes blood sugar regulation more difficult. In order to address nutritional difficulties in older people, it is essential to comprehend these changes.

Seniors frequently have a reduction in their energy requirements and a shift in their nutritional needs. While aging bodies can need fewer calories, it becomes even more important to maintain a sufficient nutrient intake. Creating nutrient-dense meals that are low in calories and high in vitamins and minerals is crucial for general health.

Older people's dietary choices may be influenced by their dental health. Potential problems that could affect chewing and food choices include dental sensitivity and tooth loss. A well-balanced and pleasurable diet can be achieved while accommodating oral problems by experimenting with different textures and opting for softer, nutrient-rich options.

The body may handle food differently in older adults due to changes in nutritional absorption and digestive problems. Including foods that are simple to digest, including cooked veggies and lean proteins, helps to maximize the absorption of nutrients and reduces the risk of an upset stomach.

Due to a reduced thirst threshold brought on by aging, older people are more vulnerable to dehydration. Maintaining adequate hydration is beneficial to kidney function and general health. Diabetes-stricken seniors should be careful how much liquid they drink, consuming water and other hydrating drinks throughout the day.

Older individuals' eating habits might be influenced by social and economic circumstances. Food quality and diversity can be impacted by a number of factors, including living alone, having little money, or having trouble getting fresh vegetables. Overcoming these obstacles is made easier by looking at practical and reasonably priced solutions while stressing nutrient-dense options.

Diabetes-afflicted seniors frequently use drugs that affect blood sugar levels. Achieving optimal glycaemic control requires synchronizing meal timing with medication regimens. An all-encompassing strategy for managing diabetes is ensured by working together with medical experts to coordinate meal planning with prescription regimens.

Dietary decisions are heavily influenced by cultural and culinary preferences. Acknowledging and honouring personal preferences enables the development of customized meal plans that complement ethnic backgrounds and culinary customs, increasing the likelihood that dietary guidelines will be followed.

Taste perception can alter with age, which may have an impact on dietary preferences. Meals are more palatable when taste alterations are addressed by experimenting with herbs, spices, and tasty seasonings. Encouraging the use of delicious and aromatic products makes eating out more enjoyable.

Encouraging social engagement among older people during mealtimes enhances their dining experience. Eating meals with loved ones, using communal eating areas, and stressing the pleasure of food not only improve the whole experience but also promote emotional health.

A personalized and nuanced strategy is necessary to address the unique dietary issues faced by older people with diabetes. People can modify their diets to support blood sugar control and foster overall well-being in later life by being aware of metabolic changes, adjusting for dental and digestive issues, and taking social, economic, and cultural variables into account.

CHAPTER THREE

PHYSICAL ACTIVITY AND DIABETES IN LATER LIFE

For seniors with diabetes, frequent physical exercise is essential to good diabetes care. Maintaining an active lifestyle becomes ever more important as people get older. This article examines the important role that exercise plays in helping seniors with diabetes. It provides information on the advantages of exercise, as well as some drawbacks and doable methods for incorporating it into daily life.

Enhancing insulin sensitivity and controlling blood sugar levels are two important benefits of physical activity. Frequent exercise improves insulin utilization in seniors with diabetes, boosting cell uptake of glucose and lowering the chance of hyperglycaemia.

Seniors frequently struggle with controlling their weight and experiencing changes in their body composition. Frequent exercise maintains weight, aids in the management of body fat, and helps maintain lean muscle mass. For seniors with diabetes, maintaining a healthy body weight is essential to overall diabetes care.

Cardiovascular problems are more likely to occur in elderly diabetics. Engaging in physical activity enhances cardiovascular health and lowers the risk of diseases like heart disease and stroke. In particular, aerobic exercises improve cardiovascular health and endurance.

Joint flexibility and health might alter with age. Stretching and low-impact workouts, which concentrate on joint mobility and flexibility, are beneficial for maintaining total joint health. This is especially advantageous for seniors with diabetes who may be prone to joint difficulties.

Sustaining balance and muscle strength is essential for avoiding falls and accidents, which can have serious repercussions for elderly people with diabetes. Weightlifting and other bodyweight exercises are examples of resistance training that help build muscle strength and improve general stability.

There is ample evidence that physical activity improves mental health. Exercise is a highly effective strategy for reducing stress, controlling anxiety, and improving mood in seniors with diabetes. Regular physical activity promotes a happy outlook and general mental well-being.

Seniors may experience problems with their sleep habits and quality. Frequent exercise improves sleep quality by easing the symptoms of insomnia and assisting in the regulation of circadian rhythms. For older people managing their diabetes and maintaining general health, better sleep quality is crucial.

Engaging in community-based physical activities or group fitness programs promotes social interaction and bonding. In addition to the physical benefits of exercise, seniors with diabetes also gain from the sense of belonging and support that comes with participating in group activities.

Seniors with diabetes should pay special attention to stress management because stress can affect blood sugar levels. Frequent exercise supports general cardiovascular health as well as the management of diabetes by lowering blood pressure and reducing stress.

It's critical for seniors to customize their fitness regimens to their specific capacities. Chair exercises, water aerobics, and low-impact activities are a few examples of workouts that can be modified to match different physical conditions and fitness levels. It is ensured that seniors can participate in regular physical exercise safely by customizing their workouts.

It is impossible to exaggerate the value of exercise for elderly people with diabetes. Frequent exercise promotes cardiovascular health, mental health, blood sugar management, and general vitality. Seniors can take charge of their diabetes care by adopting a range of exercise styles, customizing routines to meet their unique needs, and emphasizing an active lifestyle. These actions will enhance longevity and overall well-being.

Customizing Exercise Programs for Aging Bodies

Exercise regimens must be modified as people get older in order to support their general health, mobility, and well-being. Adapting exercise to older bodies is essential for seniors, especially those with diabetes, to maximize benefits and reduce the risk of injury. This article examines the value of customized exercise for senior citizens, including advice on suitable activities, safety considerations, and doable methods to maintain an active lifestyle.

Numerous physiological changes that affect muscle mass, joint health, and mobility are brought on by aging. The first step in modifying workout regimens to accommodate the unique requirements of aging bodies is acknowledging these changes. Reduced muscle mass, joint suppleness, and bone density are typical alterations.

Low-impact exercises are safer options for aging bodies and are easier on the joints. Excellent low-impact options include swimming, walking, tai chi, and stationary biking. These activities lower the risk of injuries related to high-impact exercises, enhance balance, and preserve cardiovascular health.

For aging bodies, maintaining flexibility is essential. Pilates, yoga, and stretching techniques can all help increase joint range of motion and flexibility. Incorporating these activities into a routine increases overall mobility, lowers stiffness, and helps to create a more comfortable and effective existence.

Strength training routines help older bodies maintain their muscle mass, which is a key goal. Strengthening and preserving muscle mass can be achieved by incorporating resistance training with weights, resistance bands, or bodyweight. Concentrate on addressing the main muscle groups to improve total functional ability.

Seniors must engage in balancing exercises, especially to lower their risk of falling. Balance and stability can be improved with easy exercises like heel-to-toe walking, standing on one leg, and using stability balls. Including balance training enhances general mobility and helps prevent falls.

For aging bodies, it's critical to adjust exercise intensity based on personal capacities. Gradual advancement and personalization make it safe for seniors to participate in physical exercise. A sustainable training regimen and injury prevention can be achieved by paying attention to the body's signals and avoiding undue strain.

As people age, joint health becomes increasingly important. It's critical to pay attention to these indications if joint pain or discomfort develops during or after activity. Joint-related issues can be addressed by modifying the kind or intensity of exercise, adding joint-friendly activities, and speaking with medical experts.

Elderly people may have long-term medical issues that limit their capacity to exercise, particularly if they are managing diabetes. It is ensured that exercise regimens are in line with general health objectives and any unique medical considerations by consulting with healthcare providers. Health care providers can offer advice on how to modify activities to account for medical issues.

Functional fitness is enhanced by functional movements, which replicate everyday activities. Exercises like lunges, squats, and reaching improve mobility and assist with daily duties. Including functional movements in exercise regimens helps seniors maintain their independence and participate in daily tasks more easily.

The secret to maintaining an active lifestyle is sustainability. Consistency is promoted by selecting engaging activities that suit personal interests. Finding enjoyable activities to engage in, such as dance, gardening, or group classes, can boost motivation and help make exercise a sustainable part of daily life.

Adapting exercise regimens to older bodies is a proactive way to improve general well-being and encourage healthy aging. Seniors can continue to lead active and satisfying lives by recognizing the changes that come with getting older, integrating a variety of activities, adjusting intensity levels, and placing a high priority on safety. Engaging in regular physical activity promotes mental and physical health, which in turn helps people age positively and confidently.

Breaking Through Obstacles and Including Movement in Everyday Life

Sedentary lifestyles are associated with serious health concerns, particularly for those who are managing illnesses such as diabetes. For general well-being, it is imperative to remove obstacles to physical activity and integrate movement into everyday living. This article looks at typical obstacles, doable solutions, and inventive methods to incorporate movement into everyday activities.

Comprehending the obstacles that impede physical activity is essential to formulating efficacious tactics. Lack of time, motivation, accessibility to fitness centres, health issues, and a sedentary lifestyle or employment are common obstacles. Finding individualized answers begins with acknowledging these difficulties.

Establishing reasonable and attainable objectives is essential for breaking down obstacles to physical activity. Begin with modest, doable objectives that fit your preferences and way of life. A sustainable and methodical way to integrate movement into everyday life is to gradually increase both the intensity and length of the exercise.

Maintaining an active lifestyle is much more likely to be successful when one is in a supportive atmosphere. Involve friends, family, and co-workers in the process to foster support amongst them. Accountability and motivation are enhanced by working out with a partner or engaging in group activities.

Divide up your workout into short spurts throughout the day to help you overcome the time barrier. Incorporate fast bursts of exercise, such as stretching, brisk walks, or quick workouts, while you have a break from work or are doing housework. Shorter workouts, added up over time, can be just as beneficial as a long session.

Consistent engagement is more likely when enjoyable activities are engaged in. Exercise can be enjoyable if you find things that you enjoy doing, such as dancing, gardening, swimming, or hiking. Pleasurable pursuits enable mobility to become a vital and sustainable aspect of everyday existence.

Overcoming the obstacle of a sedentary lifestyle requires a seamless integration of activity into daily chores. Use the stairs rather than the elevator, stand when conversing on the phone, or do short, easy stretches when you have a moment to spare. An increase in daily activity levels can be attributed to small, deliberate movements.

Use technology to your advantage to get past obstacles like a lack of understanding about appropriate routines or difficulty accessing fitness centres. With the help of a variety of fitness applications and internet resources, people can work out with little equipment while staying in the comfort of their own homes. Technology offers ease and flexibility.

Recognizing the importance of personal health and well-being is a powerful motivator for overcoming barriers to physical activity. Frequent exercise helps prevent and control illnesses like diabetes, so it's an investment in long-term health. Setting health first offers a strong justification for setting movement first.

Exercise should be customized to each person's ability, especially for those who are managing health concerns. To establish a customized fitness program that fits each person's ability, adaptations can include selecting low-impact workouts, adding chair exercises, or speaking with healthcare specialists.

Set aside a specific time each day for exercise and consider movement as an essential part of your life. Having a set schedule for any activity—be it walks in the morning, workouts at lunch, or night-time pursuits—increases the probability of regular adherence. Making movement a top priority increases dedication.

Removing obstacles to physical activity and integrating movement into everyday life is a life-changing path to improved health and wellbeing. People can develop a lifestyle that smoothly incorporates movement, increases vitality, and avoids the negative effects of a sedentary lifestyle by setting realistic goals, creating a supportive atmosphere, selecting fun activities, and customizing exercises to meet their needs.

CHAPTER FOUR

DRUGS AND MONITORING: A WHOLE-SYSTEM APPROACH

As people get older, controlling their diabetes becomes a more complicated and sometimes subtle undertaking. A customized strategy that takes into account age-related changes, probable comorbidities, and individual health goals is necessary for medication management, which is a critical component of diabetes care for the elderly. This article examines important factors to take into account when managing senior diabetes medications. It provides information on different medication kinds, possible problems, and ways to maximize therapy.

Physiological changes associated with aging may affect the body's reaction to diabetic drugs. Medication clearance rates can be impacted by variables such as altered metabolism and diminished renal function. Healthcare professionals must comprehend these modifications in order to choose the right drugs and dosages.

For the treatment of diabetes, a number of drug groups are frequently given; each has a distinct mode of action. Among them are:

Insulin: Seniors with diabetes are frequently prescribed insulin therapy. Different forms of insulin, such as long-acting, intermediate-acting, short-acting, and rapid-acting, offer flexibility in adjusting treatment to patient needs.

Oral Medications: Depending on the kind and severity of diabetes, doctors may give oral antidiabetic drugs such as metformin, sulfonylureas, meglitinides, and dipeptidyl peptidase-4 (DPP-4) inhibitors.

GLP-1 Receptor Agonists: To increase insulin release and lower blood sugar, injectable drugs such as glucagon-like peptide-1 (GLP-1) receptor agonists can be utilized. Compared to insulin, these drugs are given less frequently.

SGLT2 Inhibitors: Sodium-glucose cotransporter-2 (SGLT2) inhibitors are a class of drugs that limit glucose reabsorption in the kidneys, leading to increased glucose excretion in the urine.

DPP-4 Inhibitors: These drugs improve the action of incretin hormones, which stimulate insulin release and suppress glucagon secretion.

It's critical to customize drug schedules for elderly diabetics. Healthcare professionals take into account each patient's unique health status, adherence to medicine, possible adverse effects, and the existence of additional medical issues. Achieving ideal blood sugar control while lowering the chance of hypoglycaemia and other issues is the aim.

Seniors may be prescribed many medications, a phenomenon known as polypharmacy, especially if they have multiple health issues. In order to reduce the danger of polypharmacy, it is important to regularly evaluate prescriptions, simplify regimens when feasible, and make sure healthcare practitioners are communicating clearly with one another to avoid harmful interactions.

Seniors may be more vulnerable to specific undesirable reactions and side effects. It is crucial to regularly check for possible problems like hypoglycaemia, vertigo, or gastrointestinal disorders. Timely modifications to prescription regimens are made easier when seniors and healthcare practitioners communicate openly.

For elderly patients with diabetes, coordinated treatment involving multiple medical specialists is essential to drug management. For a holistic strategy, endocrinologists work with primary care physicians, pharmacists, and other specialists. Consistent communication enables modifications in response to evolving health requirements.

Medication adherence in seniors may be impacted by cognitive deterioration. Better adherence can be achieved by streamlining prescription regimens, giving clear instructions, and enlisting caregivers as needed. Changes in cognitive function are accommodated by routine follow-ups and modifications.

Dietary and activity changes are important lifestyle choices for managing diabetes. Since medication management is only one part of a holistic approach to health, healthcare providers collaborate with elders to incorporate these changes into their entire care plan.

A key component of managing diabetes is routine blood sugar monitoring. Seniors should develop a self-monitoring practice and recognize the importance of these measurements in modifying prescription dosages, with the help of healthcare practitioners.

Seniors with diabetes have unique treatment plans based on their overall health, how long they expect to live, and their preferences. Elderly patients and healthcare professionals can work together to set reasonable and attainable blood sugar control goals.

Elderly diabetes medication management necessitates a thorough and customized strategy. Seniors can manage their diabetes care with the best possible assistance by being aware of age-related changes, customizing their prescription schedules, addressing the risks associated with polypharmacy, and implementing lifestyle adjustments. Holistic diabetes treatment involves regular monitoring for any adverse effects, constant modifications, and communication with healthcare specialists. This enhances general well-being in the aging population.

Realizing the Value of Consistent Blood Sugar Monitoring

In particular, for those with diabetes, regular blood sugar monitoring is essential to managing and preserving general health. During this procedure, blood glucose levels are measured at various points during the day. For people with diabetes, it is critical to comprehend the importance of routine blood sugar monitoring because it is crucial to avoiding problems and maintaining optimal health.

People with diabetes can evaluate how effectively they are managing their condition by checking their blood sugar levels. People can better control their disease by making educated decisions about their lifestyle, medication, and nutrition by routinely monitoring their blood sugar levels. Preventing hyperglycaemia (high blood sugar) and hypoglycaemia (low blood sugar), which can both have detrimental effects on health, is essential.

Healthcare providers can better customize treatment strategies to meet the unique needs of each patient by regularly monitoring blood sugar levels. To optimize diabetes treatment, physicians can modify medication dosages, insulin dosages, or suggest lifestyle changes based on patterns and trends in blood sugar levels. This individualized strategy lowers the chance of problems and improves therapy efficacy.

A proactive approach to averting problems with diabetes is routine monitoring. Extended periods of high blood sugar might result in issues such as renal disease, nerve damage, cardiovascular illness, and eye impairment. Frequent monitoring makes it possible to identify high blood sugar early and take prompt action to reduce or eliminate the risk of severe consequences.

Sustaining stable blood glucose levels enhances one's quality of life. People with well-controlled diabetes have more energy, fewer symptoms, and are less prone to mood fluctuations. Frequent monitoring promotes a sense of control and well-being by enabling people to take ownership of their health.

A better knowledge of the ways in which many factors, including nutrition, exercise, stress, and sickness, affect blood sugar levels is fostered by monitoring blood sugar levels. People can modify their lifestyles and make educated decisions in order to better control their diabetes, thanks to this awareness. Regular monitoring also makes it easier to continue educating people about diabetes and how to manage it.

Monitoring blood sugar levels over time makes it possible to spot patterns and trends that could otherwise go missing. Both patients and medical professionals can use this information to modify treatment plans, prepare for obstacles, and avoid unexpected blood sugar rises or falls.

The foundation of successful diabetes care is routine blood sugar monitoring, which gives people the resources they need to live healthy lives. Through the provision of insightful information about blood glucose levels, people are better equipped to make educated decisions, collaborate with healthcare providers, and take preventative measures to avoid issues. For those with diabetes, making routine blood sugar monitoring a priority is essential to maintaining maximum health and wellbeing.

Working Together with Medical Experts to Adjust Medication

Effective management of diverse health disorders requires collaboration between patients and healthcare experts, particularly when it comes to medication adjustments. This cooperative approach is especially important for chronic diseases when the amount of medication needed may change over time. Better health results can be achieved by actively interacting with healthcare providers and comprehending the intricacies of this cooperation.

Effective teamwork is based on transparent and sincere communication. It should be easy for patients to talk to their healthcare providers about their symptoms, worries, and experiences. In a similar vein, healthcare professionals must foster an atmosphere that motivates patients to divulge pertinent information so that well-informed decisions can be made.

Giving a thorough medical history that includes current conditions, lifestyle choices, and any symptom changes enables medical providers to make well-informed decisions about prescribing changes. Having a comprehensive grasp of the patient's health enables customized treatment regimens that cater to each person's specific requirements.

A comprehensive knowledge of the objectives and expectations of therapy is the first step towards collaborative medication changes. Patients should talk about their goals, any adverse effects they may be having, and any aspects of their lifestyle that might affect how well they take their medications. Conversely, medical experts can shed light on the anticipated advantages and possible drawbacks of modifications.

It is essential to continuously assess general health and symptoms in order to determine whether medication adjustments are necessary. Healthcare practitioners should regularly examine the efficacy of the present pharmaceutical regimen, and patients should proactively report any changes or difficulties they encounter.

Participating actively in the decision-making process is a requirement of collaboration. Patients should be made aware of the anticipated advantages, any hazards, and the reasoning behind any suggested prescription alterations. This method of shared decision-making improves adherence to the recommended treatment plan and gives people the power to actively participate in their own healthcare.

Medical practitioners must modify a patient's pharmaceutical regimen in accordance with how well they respond to treatment. Assessing how the body is reacting to the medicine is made easier with routine check-ups, blood tests, or other pertinent evaluations. After that, changes might be made to maximize therapeutic results and reduce any possible negative effects.

Any worries or inquiries people may have regarding their prescriptions are addressed in an open discussion between patients and medical staff. Better overall health results result from this collaborative approach, which builds trust and gives patients the power to actively participate in their treatment.

Adjusting medications in conjunction with medical specialists is a dynamic and continuous procedure. Through open communication, the sharing of thorough health information, comprehension of treatment objectives, and active participation in decision-making, patients and their healthcare team can collaborate to optimize prescription regimens. To achieve and maintain excellent health in the face of changing healthcare needs, a coordinated approach is essential.

CHAPTER FIVE

EMOTIONAL WELL-BEING AND COPING MECHANISMS

Diabetes is a chronic illness that affects millions of people worldwide. It has a negative effect on emotional and physical health, especially in later life. The emotional aspects of controlling diabetes become more important as people get older. In order to provide seniors with comprehensive diabetes treatment and enhance their overall quality of life, it is imperative to acknowledge and manage the emotional burden.

In addition to the difficulties associated with managing diabetes, aging itself brings about a number of changes in life that can have a substantial impact on mental well-being. As they deal with the challenges of aging and diabetes, seniors may experience elevated levels of stress, anxiety, and even melancholy.

Medication adherence, dietary changes, and lifestyle modifications are all part of managing a chronic illness like diabetes. For seniors who may have to adjust to a different way of life in their golden years, these changes can cause feelings of frustration, loneliness, or loss.

Seniors with diabetes may worry more than usual about possible side effects such as neuropathy, cardiovascular disease, or eye problems. Stress and anxiety can be exacerbated by the dread of deteriorating health, which emphasizes the significance of attending to mental health in addition to physical health.

There is a connection between mental health and diabetes. Long-term stress can have an influence on blood sugar levels, and managing diabetes can have an impact on mental health. It's critical to identify symptoms of anxiety or depression and to get help when required in order to promote a comprehensive approach to health in later life.

Due to food restrictions, mobility challenges, or changes in lifestyle, seniors with diabetes may experience social isolation. Emotional difficulties can be made worse by loneliness, which highlights the importance of social support systems and activities that encourage social interaction.

Building a comprehensive support system is vital for seniors managing diabetes. This includes close relatives, close friends, medical experts, and support networks. Having people who are aware of the emotional elements of diabetes can be a source of support, compassion, and useful advice.

A comprehensive approach to care is necessary, given the emotional toll that diabetes takes. Seniors' emotional well-being can be greatly improved by incorporating stress-reduction strategies, counselling, and mental health assistance into diabetes treatment programs.

Seniors who are ill with diabetes need education to help them understand and manage the emotional effects of the disease. Giving people knowledge about the illness, how to manage it, and what services are available can make them feel more in control and confident about their ability to handle the challenges presented by diabetes.

The psychological effects of diabetes are a major factor in general wellbeing in later life. It is imperative that elders acknowledge and tackle these emotional obstacles in order to have satisfying lives. We can enhance the quality of life for elderly people with diabetes who are in their golden years by promoting a holistic approach that takes into account both physical and emotional health.

Establishing a Network of Support for Mental Health

Throughout life, overcoming obstacles and adjusting to changes can be difficult for one's emotional health. Creating a solid support system is essential to preserving and improving mental and emotional well-being. People can get the connections, support, and resources they need from this network to deal with the ups and downs of life. This article discusses the value of creating a support system and provides advice on how to do it for the best possible mental health.

An important aspect of general health is emotional well-being, which affects how people handle stress, manage relationships, and deal with obstacles in life. Creating a network of support is essential for developing resilience and preserving an optimistic emotional state.

Developing a support network starts with determining each person's needs. This entails considering the aspects of life—work, family, friendships, or particular difficulties like health problems or life transitions—where assistance may be helpful.

There are many different kinds of support networks, such as those made up of friends, family, mentors, co-workers, and support groups. Depending on the situation, different networks meet different needs by offering informational, practical, or emotional assistance.

Strong bonds with friends and family serve as the cornerstone of a support system. These people provide friendship, emotional understanding, and a feeling of community. By keeping lines of communication open and making time for these connections, the support system as a whole is strengthened.

Getting help from experts, like therapists or counsellors, is essential in some circumstances. These people are knowledgeable about dealing with mental health issues and can offer direction, coping mechanisms, and a secure environment for talking about private issues.

Participating in peer support groups can be especially helpful when dealing with unique issues, such as medical ailments or life transitions. These communities provide a greater understanding of one's circumstances by providing empathy, shared experiences, and a feeling of belonging.

Building supportive relationships at work is essential to stress management and emotional health maintenance. Strong relationships at work support a sense of community and offer a useful forum for talking about job-related issues.

Strong ties between people who help one another out are the foundation of a robust support system. Taking an active interest in other people's welfare reinforces the network as a whole.

In the era of digitalization, technology enables communication and connection. Social media, online forums, and virtual support networks can all be useful resources for growing and sustaining a support system, particularly in situations where geographical distances pose difficulties.

Creating a network of support needs constant work. Consistent updates, transparent correspondence, and expressing appreciation for the assistance obtained are factors that contribute to the network's longevity and efficacy.

Creating a strong support system is an investment in mental health. In times of adversity or celebration, having a network of people who support one another builds resilience and lays the groundwork for a happy and meaningful life. People can traverse life's complexity more easily and satisfactorily if they actively cultivate supportive relationships and acknowledge the significance of emotional well-being.

Diabetes Coping Techniques and Mental Health Nurturing

Living with diabetes entails more than just controlling blood sugar levels; it also calls for a comprehensive strategy that considers mental and physical health. Managing a chronic illness has an emotional cost that can affect mental health, so it's important for people with diabetes to develop psychologically resilient coping mechanisms. This article examines several methods for fostering mental wellness and managing the difficulties associated with diabetes.

Acquiring knowledge gives one strength. Being aware of the complexities of diabetes, how to manage it, and any potential problems can help people feel less anxious and more empowered to take charge of their health. A thorough understanding is enhanced by interactions with healthcare specialists, support groups, and educational materials.

A supportive atmosphere is created when feelings and concerns are shared with family, friends, and medical professionals. Maintaining mental health requires people to be able to communicate their feelings, ask for help, and create a supportive network through open communication.

Setting attainable objectives for managing diabetes can ease anxiety and increase self-assurance. Realistic goals enhance wellbeing and a sense of success, whether they involve following prescription regimens, eating a balanced diet, or exercising frequently.

Stress management techniques include yoga, deep breathing exercises, and mindfulness meditation. These methods improve general health and diabetes management by encouraging relaxation, lowering anxiety, and improving mental well-being.

One effective strategy for enhancing mental health is exercise. It improves general wellbeing, lowers stress, and releases endorphins. For people with diabetes, frequent physical activity that is tailored to their needs and preferences might be essential to maintaining their mental health.

In addition to promoting physical health, a balanced diet has a big impact on energy and mood. Healthy eating choices can have a favourable impact on mental health, and nutrition is crucial for managing diabetes.

Psychologists and counsellors are examples of mental health experts who can offer invaluable support to those managing the emotional difficulties associated with diabetes. These experts provide coping mechanisms, methods for handling stress, and a secure setting for talking about emotional issues.

Developing relationships with people who have gone through similar things can be empowering. Online forums and support groups offer a forum for advice-giving, story-sharing, and community building, which helps to lessen feelings of loneliness.

The management of diabetes requires routine blood sugar monitoring. No matter how big or small, recognizing and appreciating accomplishments helps to maintain a happy outlook. Acknowledging successes in managing diabetes increases self-esteem and one's sense of accomplishment.

Over time, diabetes management may call for modifications. It's a useful ability to be flexible and strong when faced with changes in daily schedules or treatment regimens. Having a positive view on managing the disease is enhanced by embracing flexibility.

Maintaining mental health while managing diabetes is essential to general wellbeing. People can improve their abilities to effectively handle the problems associated with diabetes, promote resilience, and lower stress levels by implementing these tactics into their daily lives. To live a happy and balanced life with diabetes, one must adopt a holistic strategy that takes into account one's mental and physical health.

CONCLUSION

When people reach their elderly years, controlling diabetes becomes crucial to preserving general health and wellbeing. It is quite feasible to not only survive but also thrive at this time of life, despite the unique hurdles presented by this chronic condition. This summary of important tactics and factors can help you live well into old age with diabetes.

Living well into old age with diabetes necessitates a comprehensive strategy that takes emotional, mental, and physical health into account. This entails adopting lifestyle habits that support a happy and healthy existence, in addition to controlling blood sugar levels.

Successful management of diabetes requires vigilant blood sugar monitoring and routine medical examinations. These procedures make it possible to identify any alterations early on, allowing for prompt modification of treatment regimens and the avoidance of consequences.

Accepting changes to one's lifestyle is essential to living well with diabetes. This entails taking up a healthy, well-balanced diet, exercising frequently, getting enough sleep, and controlling stress. These modifications improve general health in addition to controlling diabetes.

It is impossible to exaggerate the value of a support system. A foundation for emotional well-being is laid by surrounding oneself with compassionate friends, family, and medical professionals. Feelings of loneliness are lessened when there is open conversation and the sharing of experiences among community members.

Understanding is a useful tool. Taking the time to learn about diabetes, how to manage it, and the most recent developments in treatment options enables people to take an active role in their healthcare. Self-efficacy is increased, and educated decision-making is made possible by education.

Make use of technological developments in the medical field. New options for practical and effective diabetes care are provided via telemedicine services, smart devices, and continuous glucose monitoring systems. Adopting these technologies can improve the quality of life and make daily tasks simpler.

Maintaining a positive outlook is essential for living well with diabetes. Keep your optimism in the face of difficulties, celebrate your victories, and concentrate on your accomplishments. Having a happy mindset improves general wellbeing and mental toughness.

Adapting to the changes that come with aging is essential to living well with diabetes. Be adaptable to changing medical advice, lifestyle guidelines, and health requirements. Embracing change with resilience develops a proactive and empowered approach to health.

Make reasonable, attainable goals that are in line with your top priorities for your health. These objectives could include fun physical activities, maintaining a certain blood sugar target, or developing healthy eating practices. Establishing goals gives you inspiration and direction.

Lastly, enjoying each moment of life is essential to living well with diabetes. Make time for your hobbies, spend time with your loved ones, and give priority to the things that make you happy. Finding balance improves general well-being and leads to a satisfying life that extends beyond managing diabetes.

It is not only possible to thrive throughout your golden years with diabetes, but it can also result in a rich and rewarding chapter of life. People can manage the complexity of diabetes with fortitude and grace by taking a holistic approach, developing a solid support system, embracing technological improvements, keeping a positive outlook, and adapting to changes. Despite the difficulties caused by diabetes, one can, in fact, thrive, grow, and embrace life's joys during one's senior years.